MENTAL HEALTH

AND THE CRIMINAL JUSTICE SYSTEM

By Claire M. Keogh, M.A.

1

Acknowledgements

This paper was written in part-fulfilment of the Masters degree in Criminal Justice from the Institute of Public Administration, Dublin. I would like to thank the staff of the Graduate Office of the Institute of Public Administration for their support and encouragement during the course of my studies, and in particular my thesis supervisor Karen Smyth, together with my colleagues at An Garda Siochana and Shine, with whom I was working at the time. I would also like to thank my family and friends for their support and encouragement throughout my work. I would also like to thank everyone who agreed to be interviewed without whose help this dissertation would not have been possible.

TABLE OF CONTENTS

Acknowledgements...3

Table of Contents 3

Abstract..7

Definitions used in this study..8

Chapter One - Introduction 10

1.1 Introduction..10

1.2 Statement of the Problem...12

1.2 Statement of the Problem...13

1.3 Purpose of the Study 14

1.4 Research Questions...15

1.6 Theoretical Framework 16

1.7 Study Breakdown..17

Chapter Two – Literature Review..18

2.1 Introduction..18

2.2 Legislation..20

2.2 Anti – Social Behaviour and Mental Health 25

2.3 Homelessness, Mental Illness and Criminal Behaviour 27

2.4 Psychoactive drugs and competency to stand trial 31

2.5 Women in Custody and Mental Health 33

2.6 Government Policy on Mental Health 37

2.7 Concluding remarks..40

Chapter Three: Research in Other Jurisdictions 42

3.1 Introduction...42

3.2 Forensic Psychology in the UK 43

3.3 Prison Policy in UK and USA 47

3.4 Historical Context – the Victorian world view 49

3.5 Recent Developments in mental health law...50

3.6 Developments in the United States – the role of prison administrators........................52

3.7 Developments in New Zealand – non-completion of treatment 55

3.8 Concluding Comments..58

Chapter Four: Research Findings..60

4.1   Introduction 60

4.2   Limitations 61

4.3   Research Question Number One: What are the links between An Garda Siochana and the mental health services?..62

4.4   Research Question Number Two: What are the links between the courts and the Central Mental Hospital? 65

4.5   Research Question Three: The criminalisation of persons with mental illnesses 69

4.6   Research Question Number Four: What is the difference for society between retribution for a crime and rehabilitation? Does it make a difference in practice?.............72

4.7   Research Question Number Five: Discussion of competency to stand trial for mentally ill offenders; what is the role of medication in restoring competency? 75

4.8   Research Question Number Six: What about Government Policy on Mental Health, "A Vision for Change", four years after publication, in the midst of a very severe recession? 78

4.9   Concluding Comments..80

Chapter Five: Summary, Conclusions and Recommendations 82

   5.1   Summary 82

   5.2   Conclusions and Recommendations 86

References 90

Abstract

This study is about identifying and exploring the existing links between mental health and the criminal justice system. It sets out the areas of linkage between the two areas focussing on involuntary commitment, criminality in the mentally ill including courts and prisons. It refers to diversion schemes that are in place for offenders and explores the literature on the subject as well as international research in the area of mental health and criminal justice. It also exhibits the findings of nine semi-structured interviews with professionals in the field of mental health and criminal justice and carers of an offender with a mental illness.

Definitions used in this study

Mental Health Services:

This involves services which provide care and treatment to persons suffering from a mental illness or a mental disorder under the clinical direction of a consultant psychiatrist, usually in a multi-disciplinary team.

Mental Illness:

Means a state of mind of a person which affects the person's thinking, perceiving, emotion or judgement and which seriously impairs the mental function of the person to the extent that he or she requires care or medical treatment in his or her own interest or in the interest of other people (Mental Health Act 2001).

Mental Disorder:

Means mental illness, severe dementia or significant intellectual disability where—

(*a*) because of the illness, disability or dementia, there is a serious likelihood of the person concerned causing immediate and serious harm to himself or herself or to other persons, or

(*b*) (i) because of the severity of the illness, disability or dementia, the judgment of the person concerned is so impaired that failure to admit the person to an approved centre would be likely to lead to a serious deterioration in his or her condition or would prevent the administration of appropriate treatment that could be given only by such admission, and (ii) the reception, detention and treatment of the person concerned in an approved centre would be likely to benefit or alleviate the condition of that person to a material extent (Mental Health Act 2001).

Note on legal definition of mental illness:

The medical perspective of a definition of mental illness is far broader than the legal definition (Freeman, 1998). Often a legal definition refers to competency to stand trial, discussed later in the literature review. Freeman notes that a psychiatric diagnosis of a mental illness involves rigorously identifying a cluster of symptoms according to a standardised diagnostic classification system, going on to say that "a mental disorder is considered to be a group of clinically significant behaviours or patterns that cannot be an expectable response to a particular event or situation and must be considered a manifestation of a behavioural, psychological, or biological dysfunction in the person".

Chapter One - Introduction

1.1 Introduction

This study will focus on exploring the links between forensic mental health and the criminal justice system. In this regard, there will be a particular focus on the Central Mental Hospital (Central Mental Hospital) in Dundrum. The Mental Health Commission and An Garda Siochana established a working group to publish a paper which attempted to resolve certain issues of relevance in this matter. This includes the need for cooperation and alliances with mental health service users, families, and carers. In addition, a range of other disciplines may be included in the multi-disciplinary teams which provide psychiatric and social care to in-patients in mental hospitals including those charged with criminal offences who are convicted criminals or otherwise detained involuntarily. An Garda Siochana are the only criminal justice agency who are immediately available day or night to respond to crises in the community, including those involving psychiatric patients, and are often unfairly and inappropriately left to deal with mental illness and associated social crises with very limited support. The Report of the Joint Working Group on Mental Health Services and the Police (2009) was published in September 2009 and it makes a series of recommendations, some of which will be discussed in the concluding chapter to this study.

The authors of the Mental Health Commission study note that there is a dearth of research on the Irish experience in the international literature. A considerable amount of research in the field has been conducted in the USA, Canada, Australia and New Zealand, some of which will be referred to in this study. European research however is scarce.
I hope in some way to bridge the gap between the lack of data in Ireland in relation to original research in mental health and criminal justice by drawing on my own experience

within An Garda Siochana and as a volunteer in the mental health sector; and conducting interviews with various stakeholders including members of An Garda Siochana, carers of in-patients in the Central Mental Hospital, and an advocate with the Irish Advocacy Network working in forensic mental health in the Central Mental Hospital, and a social worker working in the Central Mental Hospital.

Internationally, evidence indicates increased involvement of police forces in the lives of people with mental illnesses, and this is largely due to policy changes such as deinstitutionalisation and consequent changes in treatment such as community care underpinned by the philosophy of integration in wider society. (Karem, 2005).

In 2006, the Irish government published A Vision for Change, a policy document on the future of mental health policy in Ireland. It envisaged a future of disestablishment of mental hospitals, including the disbursement of old mental hospitals and land and the reinvestment of the money into community care and social housing for mental health service users in a manner and means that the service user could access and be supported to reach their full potential as Irish citizens. It mentioned the establishment of multi-disciplinary teams for service users and care in the community. The fourth publication of the Implementation Group for A Vision for Change published recently indicates that the policy has not been fully implemented as it is under-resourced and in the current economic environment it is very difficult to find the money for increased services in the community, although Budget 2010 did make some money available for capital expenditure, this was not for services as such.

A Vision for Change makes a number of relevant recommendations in relation to forensic mental health services and court diversion schemes. This national government policy recommends that forensic mental health services should be available in all areas where law enforcement agencies are likely to encounter individuals with severe mental health problems. Recommendation 15.1.1 states that "Every person with serious mental health problems coming in to contact with the forensic system should be accorded the right of mental health care in the non-forensic mental health services unless there are cogent and legal reasons why this should not be done." (A Vision for Change, 2006)

There are many barriers to successful collaboration between police and mental health professionals. This is nowhere more evident than in the court system through which many mentally ill offenders come through to be criminalised and incarcerated and then put into the Central Mental Hospital for a time which may be longer than the prison term they may have got for what may have been a minor offence.

In this study, I will put forward the point of view of the carers of inpatients of the Central Mental Hospital. Many of these inpatients have been through the criminal justice system and have different angles on where they came into the system from a mental health background. This will be balanced by interviews with other professionals who have experience in the field and a Garda inspector and a barrister.

Cotton, 2003 notes that for the police it is their duty to protect the public and for mental health professionals it is their duty to provide treatment and care to the individual service user. He notes that members of the police force and mental health professionals have different training experiences and both work within different organisational structures which have different mechanisms of accountability.

1.2 Statement of the Problem

The purpose of this study is to investigate the links between the mental health sector and the criminal justice system. There will be a particular focus on the Central Mental Hospital in Dundrum. The insanity defence will be briefly discussed and defined. There will be a discussion the legislative process for offenders who are judged not guilty by reason of insanity or guilty with diminished responsibility who are frequently committed involuntarily to mental hospitals for punishment disguised as rehabilitation with no end date in sight.

This is an issue brought up in discussion with the carers group at the Central Mental Hospital who are attempting to bring to the attention of the relevant agencies with their interventions and discussion papers. The issue of testing of competency to stand trial in the courts system will be addressed. Competency to stand trial is a very specific type of competency, quite distinct from competency to conduct business, make wills or contracts, marry, vote or choose and refuse treatment (McGarry, 1997). Laws and courts do not allow mental patients to be generally declared incompetent for everything. The presumption of competency in all respects remains fully intact until it is successfully challenged.

Formal competency hearings occur in the criminal justice courts and very often the offender is taken to the Central Mental Hospital through the courts system or as a patient. The experience of one Garda Inspector who conducted a study recently is that a person may be taken to the Central Mental Hospital following arrest for a crime, but it is impossible to detain them involuntarily under the Mental Health Act because of the very strict criteria laid down in that Act. They may then be released to commit further crime, all the while, suffering from mental illness (Quilter, 2009).

1.3 Purpose of the Study

It has long been recognised that there is widespread community fear and misunderstanding of people who suffer from mental illness. Community attitudes concerning mentally ill offenders and their treatment by the criminal justice system are no exception (Freeman, 1998). The question of why to consider mental illness as a defence in the criminal justice system will be examined. There will also be a discussion of whether the person actually committed the unlawful act and whether there is a mental component, intent to do wrong. Did the mentally ill offender have criminal intent? Every newspaper and news television programme in recent years mentions the actions of mentally ill people in the criminal justice context of offences that have been committed. This may include what is sometimes called "murder suicides" where a person unlawfully killed a spouse and/or children before they killed themselves. In Dun Laoghaire last Christmas there was a student who was found dead with self inflicted stab wounds in the back garden after a stabbing incident in a house where his former girlfriend was seriously injured and her boyfriend also died. These crimes have become increasingly common over the last number of years.

Criminal law indicates that if an individual lacks the capacity for choice or a voluntary action it follows that under the law he or she should not be held responsible for performing a criminal act. Offenders such as these often spend significant time in the Central Mental Hospital and may be criminalised through the courts.

1.4 Research Questions

The research will focus on a number of key questions to form the main body of the dissertation. The questions will be explored in light of the literature and in light of the experience of other jurisdictions. The interviews will develop these ideas and conclusions will be drawn in the final chapter.

The questions/ discussion points are as follows:

1. What are the links between An Garda Siochana and mental health services?

2. What are the links between the courts and the Central Mental Hospital?

3. Problems with the criminalisation of mentally ill persons

4. What is the difference for society between retribution for a crime and rehabilitation, does it make a difference in practice?

5. Discussion of competency to stand trial in a mentally ill offender and what is the role of medication in restoring competency?

6. What about Government policy on mental health, "A Vision for Change" published in 2006? What has happened in relation to implementation four years on, in the depths of recession?

1.6 Theoretical Framework

This topic is one relating forensic mental health and criminal justice within a theoretical and practical framework. It will address key issues about Garda involvement in the mental health sector as they carry out duties in relation to restoring peace in society and preventing and confronting crime. The role of the Gardaí in relation to mental illness and the hospital system is that they are often the gatekeepers of the mental health system, being among the first service provider to encounter mentally ill persons in society, whether as a result of tackling crime or ensuring the safety of mentally ill persons. The theoretical framework will be based on personal observation as a Garda Civilian who has considerable voluntary experience in the mental health sector in light of the literature on the issues to be raised in this study, and original research using interviews with stakeholders working in the Central Mental Hospital such as advocates, social workers and carers, together with Garda Inspectors who are responsible for policing mentally ill persons, who may also be criminal offenders.

1.7 Study Breakdown

Chapter One – this chapter introduces the study and defines the research questions.

Chapter Two – this chapter is the review of literature set in a practical context.

Chapter Three – this chapter is a review of the international literature which discusses mental health and criminal justice in other jurisdictions.

Chapter Four – this chapter is the focus of the research to revisit the research questions. which I have undertaken referring to the semi-structured interviews with professionals and practitioners and Chief Executives working in mental health, Gardaí, a barrister, and carers.

Chapter Five – this chapter is for summary, conclusions and recommendations.

Chapter Two – Literature Review

2.1 Introduction

The focus of this study is identifying links between mental health and criminal justice and an introduction to the most common types of major mental illnesses will serve as a suitable introduction to this section of the study. Mental ill health will affect one in four people on average at some stage of their lives but many people will get over this and lead full and productive lives without ongoing treatment. Many cases of illness are much more serious than this and may be chronic or life-long in nature. The most common types of mental illnesses associated with criminal behaviour would be illnesses such as schizophrenia, bipolar disorder and schizo-affective disorder. Schizophrenia is an illness of the mind developed by 1% of the world's population and it can lead to delusions, false beliefs, paranoia, disorganised thinking and socially dysfunctional behaviours. Bipolar disorder is a mood disorder also experienced by 1% of the world's population and it can lead to highs and lows of mood in a sufferer. They can experience mania or deep depression and can also exhibit symptoms of delusions or false beliefs. Schizo-affective disorder is experienced by one in two hundred people and sufferers exhibit symptoms of both schizophrenia and bipolar disorder (The Schizophrenia Handbook, 2004).

The hearing of voices in one's head is a feature of each of these types of illnesses and this is commonly what leads a person with a mental illness to commit serious crime while they are having an acute episode of illness. In Irish legislation there have been a number of acts of legislation which impact on people with mental illnesses during their time either as a patient in a hospital, or during incarceration while they are awaiting trial. These acts are discussed below.

2.2 Legislation

Mental Health Act 2001

Definitions from the Act relating to mental illness and mental disorder precede this study. The Act provides for the involuntary admission to 'approved centres' for persons suffering from mental disorders. It provides for the independent review of the involuntary admission of such persons by a tribunal. It also serves to repeal the Mental Treatment Act 1945. The Central Mental Hospital (Central Mental Hospital) is among the approved centres provided for under this Act (Kennedy, 2007). In terms of criminal justice the role of the Gardaí in relation to involuntary admissions under the Mental Health Act is a very significant matter for the families involved and the mental health service users themselves because of the perception that Gardaí are only involved in arresting people for criminal behaviour.

Focus groups recently facilitated by Shine, the organisation that upholds and supports all those affected by mental ill health, have highlighted the experience that frequently an involuntary admission involving the attendance of the Gardaí has all the elements of arrest. Furthermore, in most cases there is virtually no therapeutic element involved in the process of getting the person into hospital. Issues raised in focus groups include the inappropriate use of excessive restraint, handcuffs and marked cars outside the house are reported (Shine, 2009). Having said this many families do speak positively of the involvement of the Gardaí during involuntary admission. And Director of Shine has noted to me in a 2009 interview that things are much better in these instances since the Mental Health Act 2001 was enacted. The Mental Health Act 2001 provides for the role of the Authorised Officer and this has the potential to have a significant and positive impact in these situations. The authorised officer and Gardaí must work together as a team to ensure sensitive and supportive process for the service user and family involved (Kennedy). Prior to that there was the 1945 Act and it involved a Garda escorting a person to hospital in most instances during involuntary hospitalisations.

The unavailability of community mental health services or crisis outreach services means that when a person with a mental illness reaches crisis point, involuntary admission is the only option. Many Gardaí with little training in mental health may find themselves in a family home, trying to work with a person who has not committed any crime, but who, they may assume will present a significant threat. In recent years Garda recruits have received training in mental health during their two years in training, but older Gardaí may not have the training beyond the legislation itself. Also, there is a very significant stigma attached to mental illness within the family of a person with a mental illness and this is compounded when involuntary admissions under the Mental Health Act 2001 happen.

The Criminal Law (Insanity) Act 2006

This Act was passed to amend the law relating to unfitness to plead in a criminal trial and to replace the special verdict of guilty but insane, with not guilty by reason of insanity. This Act is involved with the trial and detention of persons suffering from mental disorders who are charged with offences. This Act provides for the committal of such persons to 'designated centres' and for the independent review of the detention of such persons. It also established the Mental Health Criminal Law Review Board. It must be noted that approved centres as defined in the Mental Health Act 2001 and the designated centres provided for in the Criminal Law (Insanity) Act 2006 are different. The distinction may raise the possibility of discrimination.

The European Convention of Human Rights (ECHR) Article 14 prohibits discrimination. In a judgement of the European Court of Human Rights, Pretty Vs. UK, 2002, there was a stated principle that "for the purposes of Article 14 a difference in treatment between persons in an analogous or relevantly similar positions is discriminatory if there is no objective and reasonable justification…Discrimination may also arise where states without an objective and reasonable justification fail to treat differently persons whose situations are significantly different" (Kennedy, 2007). In this manner criminal offenders with mental illnesses can justifiably be treated differently from mental patients involuntarily admitted under the Mental Health Act 2001 who have not committed a crime. Also, these differences are clearly defined procedurally and legally, however he notes that some people with mental illnesses end up in prisons. In addition, in fact, in the Central Mental Hospital, among the 82 patients residing there, many have been kept involuntarily for many years, going back to before the Mental Health Act of 2001, and to the families and carers of those persons, there is very little difference in the way their loved ones are treated and the treatment of criminals who have been convicted through the courts.

The Criminal Law Insanity Act 2006 does not require the court to hear evidence from a psychiatrist or any other witness whether expert or not, before making a determination concerning fitness to be tried. However, appeals can arise from the evidence of a psychiatrist. Kennedy, 2007, notes that any court of first instance would be unwise to make a finding of unfitness without supporting evidence from a psychiatrist. The Act provides that having made a determination that the accused is unfit to be tried, evidence can be heard as to whether or not the accused did the alleged act and if there is a reasonable doubt, the accused should be discharged.

A discussion of forensic commitments will follow in Chapter Four in the semi-structured interviews with professionals working in the Central Mental Hospital. With commitment to the Central Mental Hospital we know that instead of being jailed many persons charged with criminal offences are hospitalised involuntarily there. Some forensic patients await a determination of their competency to stand trial; others are being treated for restoration to such competency and those who are extremely impaired have little prospect of restoration to either competency or liberty. Many patients in the Central Mental Hospital were tried and found not guilty by reason of insanity at the time of their crimes. They are involuntarily institutionalised even though found "innocent" according to a court of law. In an American context, Edwards notes that in many cases "[they] spend more time in a psychiatric institution than they would have served in prison had they been found guilty" (Edwards, 1998).

Upon release from prison, or involuntary hospitalisation, **homelessness** often becomes an issue for a significant number patients or criminal offenders. **Anti-social behaviour** can often become a problem for people such as these and these factors and how they impact on people with mental illnesses will be discussed in the next sections of this chapter.

2.2 Anti – Social Behaviour and Mental Health

In the United Kingdom in 1999, Tony Blair's government introduced Anti Social Behaviour Orders (ASBOS), which the police and courts have had regard to for over the last decade. They are intended to be a low-level response to public nuisance type incidents such as public order offences which can be administered to any person over the age of ten who commits an offence. These types of instruments for dealing with public order offences and minor crimes are also now available to Gardaí in the Irish context. These orders can have a profoundly negative impact on people with mental illnesses. The ASBO itself is a civil tool; however a breach of its terms leads to immediate legal repercussions, which can lead to five years imprisonment (Connolly, 2005). This can have a significant impact on a person suffering from a mental disorder, within the meaning of the Mental Health Act, 2001. A person suffering from mental ill health may not be fully aware of the impact of their own behaviour and could fail to recognise or understand the legal implications of non-compliance with ASBO terms. This leads to the criminalisation of a person who is unwell for sometimes very minor offences. It could be argued that this significantly at odds with any notion of a therapeutic response to mental illness in the community or of a rights-based society that promotes equality for all.

Edwards, 1998 notes that there are significant differences between punishing convicted criminals in penal institutions and treating those acquitted of crimes committed because of insanity. Convicted criminals are punished for several reasons: to prevent and deter similar offences; to rehabilitate and to extract retribution for society for the crimes committed. Mental institutions, he further notes, also offer prevention and deterrence and rehabilitation but they differ in theory from penal institutions in that it is improper to use them to extract societal "revenge". In practice, however there is often little difference between the two in any of these respects, and in the Irish context at least, revenge is a word not often found in the literature and it does not coincide easily with the work of rehabilitation that is apparently going on inside mental institutions such as the Central Mental Hospital.

2.3 Homelessness, Mental Illness and Criminal Behaviour

People who work with the mentally ill or the homeless will have first hand evidence of persons being criminalised as a result of their circumstances. In this regard being mentally ill and/or homeless may have led to criminal behaviour. Focus Ireland note in a 2007 report that numerous studies suggest that being homeless increases significantly the chances of individuals entering the criminal justice system. For example the Crime and Homelessness Study in 2002 shows that the relationship between homelessness and crime is a complex one. For less than half the sample being homeless led to a crime which in turn led to imprisonment. For others it was being released from prison that led directly to homelessness. The study notes that the types of crime committed by those homeless prior to first being imprisoned is commonly larceny, vagrancy and drugs offences. In contrast, people homeless following release from prison commit much more "serious" crime (Hickey, 2002). In determining the relationship between crime and homelessness a key question relates to whether homelessness leads to offending or vice versa. Research seems to suggest that crime can both be a cause and an effect of homelessness and it is important to note that risk factors and triggers associated with homelessness can often underlie the offending behaviour (Focus Ireland 2007).

People who experience homelessness are more likely than other people to have a mental illness, and this is well documented both in European and American research studies. These studies suggest that homeless adults may be twice as likely as the general population to have a mental illness, with Feeney et al, 2000, estimating that between 25 and 50 percent have severe psychiatric disorders. In research conducted among hostel dwelling men in Dublin, this has been confirmed, with findings that 64 percent were suffering from some form of mental health condition (Feeney et al, 2000).

Case management

The Gardaí work closely with the Homeless Agency in relation to case management for offenders who are homeless or at risk of homelessness and have entered the criminal justice system. A pilot project regarding case management for young criminal offenders took place in Dublin's North Central Division in 2006 (Feehan and Brown, 2009). This project began in an attempt to deal with the increasing problem of young people in conflict with the law. The process places one Garda as a Case Manager for each individual young person with the aim of leading, co-ordinating and managing the young person's charges. The project also aims to involve the case manager closely with the young person, their family and all the agencies that may be involved in the hope of improving the outcomes for the young person. This project has proved very successful and An Garda Siochana is in the process of implementing case management nationwide. This will be developed further in Chapter Four in an interview with a Garda Inspector.

Diverting young people out of the criminal justice system or reducing the numbers of criminal offences they have through case management will also have an ancillary impact on mentally ill offenders who are diverted through the mental health system. Case management is a process designed by An Garda Siochana to manage the criminal behaviour of juveniles, but some of these juveniles have aged out having turned eighteen years old, and some may be at risk of homelessness or have mental health problems as a result of a difficult background. However, offenders identified as having mental illnesses must be taken to Central Mental Hospital through the courts system before diversionary process can begin and this again has the effect of criminalising the mentally ill, an issue which will be discussed with carers in Chapter Four of this study. It is noted that case management only happens with young people who have a history of criminal offences, first time offenders would not be case managed.

Many of the young people who do age out may end up in the psychiatric services and on medication for various disorders variously described as mental illness. This may be a few years after they have aged out sometimes in their mid-twenties. Psychoactive drug therapy will be discussed in the next section.

2.4 Psychoactive drugs and competency to stand trial

Psychoactive drugs are usually prescribed to restore competency to stand trial and to enable mentally ill offenders recover normal brain activity following a psychotic episode during which time they have committed offences and have come to the attention of the Gardaí, often for very serious crimes and very violent attacks. Within the Irish context, a prisoner, in tandem with all other mentally ill citizens, has a right to refuse such treatment if they do not give consent. But this is a very grey area, because if they are deemed to be unable to give consent by reason of being mentally ill, then treatment may be prescribed and administered in the best interests of the patient, albeit involuntarily. Some courts and legal authorities in the international context champion a right not to be drugged to stand trial (Edwards, 1998).

The medical model, which is used in many western countries including Ireland, indicates that the treatment of choice for mentally ill persons is drug therapy using psychoactive drugs. Sometimes this is in conjunction with talk therapy or counselling but in the Irish context; there are usually very long waiting lists in the community for such therapy for most individuals. For the eighty-two patients of the Central Mental Hospital however, multi-disciplinary consultant-led teams including psychologists and counsellors are onsite and available for in-patients rehabilitation purposes, both for those committed involuntarily through the criminal justice system and those serving sentences that are too ill for jails. Despite the efficacy of psychoactive drugs, chemical competency to stand trial is vigorously contested by the various stakeholders in the criminal justice system. Some proponents of drug therapy find the very idea of chemical competency to stand trial abhorrent, unaware perhaps that ordinary competence depends upon normal brain chemistry and that drug therapy can facilitate a return towards normal brain chemistry (Edwards, 1998).

In my experience people with major mental illnesses such as schizophrenia and bipolar disorder can be very well managed on medication and can lead very successful lives; and the numbers of mentally ill persons who engage in criminality is surprisingly small. As Edwards (1998) notes, if properly used, psychoactive drugs can help restore memory, a sense of personal identity and varying degrees of rational capacity. This is typically what happens during drug therapy, both within and outside of the criminal justice system in the psychiatric services.

So far in this chapter, I have discussed types of mental illnesses, legislation, and the impact of homelessness and anti-social behaviour on criminal offenders or persons with mental illnesses. I have also discussed drug therapy. The next section will focus on the ways in which the criminal justice experience differs for women with mental illnesses, who are in the minority in the prison population, but who may have proportionately more mental illness than the same cohort of male prisoners.

2.5 Women in Custody and Mental Health

Women make up about five per cent of prison populations worldwide (Stern, 1998) and this is also true in the Irish context. Much of the research that has been carried out has been focussed on male prisoners as a result, the majority of the prison population. However a minority status and marginalisation increases the need to recognise women in prison and indeed in mental hospitals as a distinct group with distinctive needs. Women with mental illnesses are further marginalised. A consistent picture of poverty, marginalisation, victimisation and deprivation makes up the basis of every female custodial population in every jurisdiction (Loucks, 2004). Many women who do end up in custody have backgrounds which feature such difficulties as drug addiction, abuse, poverty and unemployment together with psychological disturbance which may be described as mental illnesses. Many of these women go from the Dochas Centre in Mountjoy to the Central Mental Hospital in Dundrum depending on the circumstances. This pattern is not exclusive to women, but it does characterise a large number of women in the prison or mental hospital population, (example Byrne and Howells, 2002, quoted in Loucks, 2004 in a Scottish context).

Loucks conducted research in 1998 and a recurrent theme throughout her research into women in custody is the finding that so many of the women are victims as well as offenders. In Scotland the vast majority of women in prison had been direct or indirect victims of sexual or emotional or physical abuse and often a combination of these. Most women who reported being victims of abuse said this had taken place at many times throughout their lives, often as children, teenagers and as adults. Many women in custody reported going back out to violent families or partners and for some, prison was the first safe place they had been (Loucks,

2004).   I would note here that some research appears to show that women who have been abused as young people also find partners who abuse them and they end up in a cycle of abuse, often choosing the wrong partners or spouses and feeling trapped and unable to leave due to economic circumstances, family circumstances, addiction problems and unemployment.

Suicide and self-injury as a result of mental illness are common experiences for a significant proportion of female prisoners. However, suicide attempts are more common outside custody within the community than in prisons or mental hospitals. In the last month (August 2010) a female prisoner in the Dochas Centre took her own life. She was serving life in jail for drowning her only son. In the Scottish study, only seven of the twenty-nine women who had said they had tried to kill themselves had tried it while in custody. Research in England and Wales shows that forty percent of women in custody had received help or treatment for a mental health or emotional problem in the year before they entered custody. This was double the proportion of male prisoners (Singleton et al, 1998). They note that women in prison prior to conviction or sentence contain the highest proportion of prisoners ever admitted to a psychiatric hospital at 22%, including 6% admitted for six months or more and 11% admitted to a secure ward. Loucks notes that this compares to 8% of male prisoners with 2% admitted for six months or more and 3% in a secure facility. In an Irish context, a recent study by a team led by the Clinical Director of the Central Mental Hospital revealed that 60 per cent of female prisoners and 35 per cent of male prisoners have experienced a mental illness at some stage in their lives and criticised the use of prisons as "psychiatric waiting rooms" (Duffy et al, 2006).

Psychological distress is the common feature of women in custody, particularly in light of their extensive histories of suicidal behaviour, mental health problems, addiction and abuse. On the Beck Hopelessness Scale (Beck et al, 1974), the research shows that there are clinical levels of hopelessness for a high proportion of women in custody. Prisoners often score highly for hopelessness using this scale. Samber and Porporino, 1998, found for example that a third of their subjects scored six or higher out of twenty, where higher scores indicate a greater level of hopelessness. In Scotland, the average score for women in prison was 6.3 (Loucks, 2004).

According to Singleton et al 1998, 59% of remand male prisoners and 40% of sentenced male prisoners were assessed as having a neurotic disorder. The proportions for women were 76% of remand prisoners and 63% of sentenced female prisoners. These were commonly mixed anxiety and depressive disorders. Psychotic disorders may be more common among female prisoners on remand, 21% as assessed by lay interviews as compared to 9% of male remand prisoners.

Women are allowed have young babies in the Dochas centre live with them until they are nearly two years old, but the separation after this time must be a source of considerable mental distress. Separation from children and families appears to be a bigger problem for female prisoners than male prisoners. In families where the woman is in custody and there are children to be looked after, research shows that they are much less likely to be looked after by the other parent, than they are if the father is in prison to be looked after by the mother. Research in Scotland by the Inspectorate of Prisons and Social Work Services 1998 found that 17% of fathers looked after their children while the mother was in custody and this compares to 87% of mothers who cared for the children while the father was in prison.

A common feature of female prisoners is that they are drawn from a group who share all the characteristics of social exclusion. Mentally ill female prisoners are even more socially excluded than the rest. What this means for social policy and what specifically is government policy on mental health will be discussed in the next section of this chapter.

2.6 Government Policy on Mental Health

In January 2006, the Government adopted the Report of the Expert Group on Mental Health Policy **"A Vision for Change"** as the basis for the future of the mental health services in Ireland. In March 2006, the then Minister for State at the Department of Health and Children Mr. Tim O'Malley with special responsibility for mental health services established in Independent Monitoring Group for three year progress period, to monitor progress on the implementation of the report recommendations.

In June 2010, the Fourth Annual Report on Implementation of "A Vision for Change" was published. The Independent Monitoring Group notes that the HSE is currently developing a proposal and a business case for the development of a new central mental hospital. This proposal will also enable a decision on the location to be finalised. In recent years the proposed relocation of the Central Mental Hospital in Dundrum has caused considerable difficulty for service providers working with the mentally ill in Ireland because of the suggestion that it should be located in the grounds of the new "super-prison" which is to be located at Thornton Hall.

The organisations who work on behalf of mental health service users will note that there is already a significant stigma attached to having a mental illness. Having a central mental hospital located on a prison site reinforces the stigma and seems to criminalise the mentally ill, regardless of whether or not they have a criminal background. It seems to blur the distinction between involuntary commitment and incarceration, a topic which will be explored further in Chapter Four in interviews with professionals working in the field. In the public's mind, who may not have much experience or knowledge about these matters, and rely on the media for commentary (which may be biased), the mentally ill will be placed in the same category as criminal offenders.

When "A Vision for Change" was published in 2006 money appeared to be no object for the Government who had large surplus funds to work with for a number of years up until that time. In the document was a plan to sell off old mental hospitals and replace this with the concept of care in the community, using the funds from institutions sales to fund the of purchase social housing for the mentally ill in the community who would be supported to live independently. They would be cared for by consultant-led multi-disciplinary teams within the community. Four years on, this plan has not been implemented.

In recent years inspections of mental hospitals have found that many of them are not fit for habitation, (eg. St. Brendans, St. Ita's). These hospitals were inspected earlier in 2010 and earmarked for closure to new patients. A policy of closing old hospitals that are full of institutionalised patients has begun and the community-based care or supported social housing has not yet been funded by the Government. The patients end up losing the stability they have grown accustomed to, albeit institutionalised care in old hospitals, and they end up moving to new wings of general hospitals where the care may not be much better. There have been cuts to the portion of the healthcare budget earmarked for mental health since the start of the recession and as we face into Budget 2011 where another €3Billion of cuts will have to take place, this will inevitably involve cuts to the healthcare budget which accounts for a third of total government spending.

As mentioned earlier, homelessness becomes an inevitable issue for many mentally ill people who are released from hospitals. In relation to mental health services for homeless people, the

Report of the Independent Monitoring Group states that of the five recommendations in "A Vision for Change" only one has been partially implemented to date. All through the report they note progress that has only been partial or not implemented at all. The authors recommend that the plan should be fully implemented in the original timeframe of 7-10 years. Four years on from publication, and two years into a deep recession, the prospects for full implementation look grim.

2.7 Concluding remarks

In this literature review, I have introduced the types of major mental illnesses which may lead people to commit crime in the first place, 'hearing voices' for example.

I would also note here that contrary to bias in the media against people with mental illnesses, the number of people with mental illnesses who do commit crime is relatively small. In my experience of working within Shine in a voluntary capacity in recent years, I can count on one hand the number of people I have met who have mentioned having a criminal record. Comments in interviews from relevant professionals conducted during this study reinforce this view.

I have introduced summaries of the major pieces of legislation to be passed in the last ten years affecting people with mental illnesses, and that portion of people with mental illnesses who commit crime.

I have also reflected on issues of homelessness of mentally ill persons and the impact of that on criminal behaviour. I have reflected on anti-social behaviour and the process of criminalising the mentally ill for what may be minor offences and the questions that arise out of that.

I have spoken about psychiatric medication in the 'medical model' and its role in caring for the general population of persons with mental illnesses in addition to the special role of drug therapy in relation to treatment of criminal offenders awaiting trial.

I have reflected on the special circumstances which gender differences play in the care of women prisoners with mental illnesses, including a background of marginalisation and social exclusion felt by many.

Chapter 3 will draw on international research into the issues linking mental health to the criminal justice system as distinct from what has essentially been a review of the literature in an Irish context. Some of the conclusions that are drawn in the studies may be relevant to mental health and criminal justice as a whole, not just within the context in which the study took place.

Chapter Three: Research in Other Jurisdictions

3.1 Introduction

The review of the literature in the previous chapter indicates that there are quite a number of areas in this complex topic linking mental health to the criminal justice system. In this chapter I will attempt to refer to the research in other jurisdictions in relation to this. An introduction to forensic psychology from a United Kingdom perspective will constitute the first section of the chapter. This will be followed by a brief overview of prison policy in the United Kingdom and the United States. Then, the historical backdrop of mental health in the Victorian era will be discussed in relation to how institutionalisation of mental patients developed, followed by an exploration of the legalism which followed this period. The role of prison administrators in the US in relation to committing offenders to mental health institutions will be discussed next and the impact on personal liberty and human rights law. Finally, there will be a discussion of treatment non-completion in Queensland, which forms part of a New Zealand study. Finally, I will summarise the key points in the concluding section to the chapter.

3.2 Forensic Psychology in the UK

Writing in the UK, Adler (2004) notes that in many parts of the world today it is possible to find psychology being practiced with a forensic twist. She notes that forensic psychologists evaluate offender behaviour programmes, design risk assessments and investigative processes, support victims, provide treatment and generally try to facilitate justice. As such psychological testing is now fairly commonplace within the courts themselves.

Dushkind (1984) notes that most people would say that forensic psychology is concerned with providing psychological information to people agencies and systems involved directly and sometimes indirectly with the implementation of justice. Sometimes forensic psychology is defined more narrowly as work carried out for use solely by the court. This definition is based on a literal reading of the word forensic, but in the UK at least this is not the definition most usually adopted or practiced. In much of Europe, the relationship between criminality and psychology has been strengthened in recent years with the growth of effective practice initiatives (Adler, 2004). Applied psychology has generally expanded and given greater credence to sociological theories.

In the foreword to the third edition of the Oxford Handbook of Criminology, there is an acknowledgement that 'in recent years psychological approaches to crime had become increasingly prominent in both academic and public policy' (Maguire, Morgan and Reiner, 2002). One area in which forensic psychologists have been active alongside people working in related disciplines is in designing and evaluating programmes targeted at reducing recidivism, often in violent, sexual and or mentally disordered offenders (Adler, 2004). Alongside this work much effort has been expended on risk assessments, both on their design and conduct. In England and Wales, as elsewhere, the merits of different sorts of risk assessment are not only a source of contention but a good example of how psychological tools may be used by legislative authorities. There is a history for example of psycho-legal involvement in dealing with or disposing of the mentally or personality-disordered offender, and there have been ongoing attempts over many years to update the UK Mental Health Act 1983. Bell et al, 2003, note that **dangerous and severely personality disordered** (DSPD) is not a clinical diagnosis. They say it is a policy inspired label that describes the few disordered people who suffer from a severe personality disorder and because of their disorder they pose a significant risk of serious harm to others.

Adler (2004) notes that the DSPD policy is a partial replacement for the 'psychopathic' label, although the two are by no means the same. Psychopathy is a legal concept defined within the Mental Health Act of 1983 and within that legislative description is the notion of 'persistent and untreatable behaviour'. She notes that when applied by the criminal justice system, a label of psychopathy for an individual could result in an indeterminate stay in a special hospital or high security facility for offenders with serious psychiatric and psychological problems. This debate going on in England and Wales is also one that goes on in Ireland in relation to patients in the Central Mental Hospital who go between prison and the hospital, some of whom serve out life sentences in the Central Mental Hospital.

It is a deeply felt and much argued debate whether psychopathic offenders are able to benefit from a stay in a psychiatric hospital. Adler points out that some would say they are untreatable by definition so they should be incarcerated in prisons on the basis of their offending behaviour alone. This is a debate that touches on fundamentals of psychology, psychiatry and treatment. There are also human rights implications as a stay in a special hospital is usually of indeterminate length, often resulting in a longer period of confinement than a normal corresponding period of incarceration in prison.

In England and Wales, the literature notes that psychopathic offenders have been held both in prisons and in special hospitals alike. Perkins and Bishop 2003, UK academics, have noted that in practice DSPD might be seen as 'an attempt to quantify a distinction between the general category of mentally disordered offenders and an extreme subgroup whose disorder is manifested in the kinds of extreme violence and sexual aggression that has caused most public concern.'

In my view there is a very serious distinction to be drawn between mentally disordered offenders who have a diagnosable mental illness such as schizophrenia, and the type of violent personality disordered offender mentioned here. In Chapter Four in my interviews of professionals it will be noted that the large majority of people with the most common types of mental illnesses who come to the attention of An Garda Siochana do so with minor public order offences as a result of what may be voices in their head or muddled or disorganised thinking.

Bell et al, 2003 note that to be in the special subgroup of mentally disordered offenders a person must demonstrate a high level of personality disorder, be more likely than not to offend seriously, and crucially there must be a functional link between these two. These policies are already being implemented, Adler notes, but there are still major issues of definition and practice to be resolved and legislation has yet to be brought before the UK Houses of Parliament.

There are questions about how to measure the entry criteria and define someone as DSPD in the first place, but what would be the criteria for release or for transmission to a less secure environment. Perkins and Bishop 2003 have raised this question alongside a useful consideration of the very nature of dangerousness and the conceptualisation of personality and personality disorder.

Comparing to the Irish context it is noted in Chapter Four that the Criminal Law Insanity Act 2006 which provides for persons to be found not guilty by reason of insanity and detained in the Central Mental Hospital. This legislation does not allow for conditions to be set upon release from Central Mental Hospital and as such the small numbers of people found not guilty by reason of insanity since the enactment of the act have therefore never been released at all because amendments to the Act providing for conditional discharge have not gone through the Oireachtas as yet. However, a review board does meet every six months to review each case.

The carers group for example at the Central Mental Hospital have been instrumental at driving this and they hope these amendments will be through before the end of this year (2010).

3.3 Prison Policy in UK and USA

In North America much of Europe's modern prison policies have been characterised by swings from rehabilitative to punitive measures and back again. Essentially, what is the prime purpose of imprisonment, how can we assess whether its goals have been met, and does it disproportionately affect some more than others. In the UK context, Melossi (2000) observes how public attitudes towards offenders may fluctuate with social and economic conditions. In certain societal periods, criminals, some of them at least, have been considered more as innovators and heroes than villains and rates of imprisonment decline accordingly. Other times, largely due to social construction by agents of a normative order, the criminal becomes the villain, a public enemy, and becomes more repugnant to authority and public alike. At these times, the use of imprisonment rises. A defining feature of these intermittent social conditions seems to be financial prosperity. As the economy flourishes, the use of imprisonment falls and as economic conditions deteriorate so the use of imprisonment rises (eg. Chiricos and Delone 1992 and Melossi 2000). Melossi is writing in the UK context and Chiricos and Delone are writing in the US context but the research appears to say the same thing.

Writing in the UK, Sparks (2000) adds to the above economic paradigm by explaining how peoples attitudes to punishment may be shaped by the 'doctrine of less eligibility' which is essentially the notion that prison conditions must be worse than the living conditions of the working poor in that society. He argues that during time of high unemployment members of the public expect prison conditions to be more austere than the conditions endured by the poorest members of society. In an Eastern European context, Kury and Ferdinand (1999) observe that members of the public in Eastern European countries became more punitive in their attitudes to offenders during the social uncertainties brought about by the demise of the communist regime. From a sociological perspective it seems reasonable to assume that public attitudes to crime and justice may reflect socio-economic dynamics of a given culture. Consequently, attempts to assess attitudes may not always yield a consistently accurate measure of public beliefs.

The topic and scope of this dissertation identifying links between mental health and the criminal justice system does not allow for an extensive discussion on public attitudes to general prison confinement, rather it involves the determination of whether or not the 'departure from sound mind be of a nature to justify the confinement of the individual' (question raised by nineteenth century medic John Connolly). He concluded that such enquires were likely to show that 'complete restraint is very rarely required' (quoted in Schull, 1985, p129). In 19th century language complete restraint might mean compulsory or involuntary admission.

3.4 Historical Context – the Victorian world view

There have always been questions about the justifications for detention in a mental hospital including how best to secure the patients rights and defining the duties of those doing the detaining. This dilemma has been around for centuries and perhaps those who agonised most over these questions were the Victorians as Philip Bean notes (2008). He says their instincts towards liberty supported leaving alone the mad and eccentrics but their therapeutic and paternalistic ethics urged them to help (quoted in Porter, 1991). The Victorians sought to resolve their dilemma through legalism legislation aimed at providing the courts with powers to decide on admissions while restricting the asylum managers and those conducting treatment. Bean notes, that in the UK context each facet of the patients' life and treatment was controlled according to a detailed set of rights and duties imposed on patients and staff alike, based on the assumption that no person ought to be confined without legal safeguards. There were deeply held suspicions of those claiming expertise on ability to diagnose and treat the insane which supported their beliefs.

This Victorian way of thinking about mental illness and confinement continued throughout the first half of the last century, and was not only confined to the UK. Questions about the quality and the veracity of treatments, the reliability of diagnoses and the fear that mental illness could be confused with anti social behaviour were regular features of psychiatric literature. As late as 1960 the British Medical Journal agonised about the difference between social misdemeanour and mental illness, after a young man, apparently resistant to the crime and punishment formula of the courts was handed over to psychiatrists for a leucotomy. In the subsequent correspondence one doctor thought it was indeed fortunate that this procedure was not practiced one hundred years earlier, otherwise Dostoevsky might well have been a candidate and the world would never have his insightful literature.

3.5 Recent Developments in mental health law

In modern times the law has become the vehicle by which treatment and therapy are advanced, not the means by which the treatment provider can be controlled. Detention has become the prerogative of the medical profession and as Peay (2003) points out, mental health law is now largely applied by non-lawyers. Members of that profession, not the courts are given the primary responsibility and the powers to decide who should and who should not be admitted and the treatment to be provided. The courts retain limited powers but there are fewer checks and balances than before. In the Irish context, mental health tribunals have been introduced with the Mental Health Act 2001 and a patient would have a legal representative to determine if a period of involuntary admission could be extended in accordance with law.

Times have changed since legalism and the knowledge, prestige and powers of modern medicine have accompanied those changes, often to the benefit of the patient but not always so (Bean 2008). Most jurisdictions have done away with Victorian asylums to be replaced with modern buildings where the mentally ill are treated to modern methods of medical care. This involves new forms of treatment replacing older ones that may be painful and degrading although some would say that modern treatments are no more effective (Kerr, 1983). In my opinion modern pharmacological treatments have been nothing short of revolutionary as when they are effective and a patient is compliant they can often lead full and productive lives with only very short and intermittent periods of ill health. Mental patients may benefit from standards of care beyond the dreams of our Victorian forebears whether they are of comfortable surroundings or modern chemical medications; they are markedly different experience from earlier robust forms of treatment, such as psycho-surgery or electric shock treatment. Electro-convulsive therapy (ECT) is still sometimes practised in this jurisdiction and others for particularly severe cases of mental illness that are resistant to modern drug treatment but there are legal safeguards for the patient regarding consent. Attempts have been made to outlaw the practice in some jurisdictions including New Zealand, Australia and the USA and the practice of it is generally declining.

Modern health legislation is characterised by looking towards the rights and privileges of professionals not backwards towards the imposition of duties. The law is likely to have only a limited impact unless it is countered with the values of those who use it, and it must reflect the ethics of healthcare to encourage rather than to deter good practice (Expert Committee, 1999). The Expert Committee also say that the more in tune any new legislation is with the aspirations of those who have to use it the more it will be followed in practice. Notably, the aspirations of the patients are not mentioned.

Civil commitment statutes in most jurisdictions include three conditions for involuntary commitment. This is also the case in Ireland. These conditions are the mental disorder itself, the need to protect others and the need to protect oneself. Some commentators such as US based Thomas Szasz argue that these conditions have never provided adequate justification for commitment, for he is convinced that mental illness is a myth and hospitalisation is a modern form of state controlled warfare (Szasz, 1960). His critics say that such views ignore the reality of mental disorder, the agonising and the hardship both in the patient and in the family of what can be a very painful condition that has a drastic impact on quality of life for those affected. Of the three conditions the first and most important is the mental disorder although mental disorder alone is not sufficient to justify compulsory detention. Most psychiatrists would however view a serious mental disorder as by definition sufficient to require protection for the patient, or for others, or for both.

3.6 Developments in the United States – the role of prison administrators

In the context of the United States we see similar types of questions being raised and research conducted on similar topics as jurisdictions closer to home such as the UK and Ireland. Thomas Look for example, writing in the US in 1978, notes that prison administrators have historically exercised what many legal scholars characterise as autocratic discretion. The transfer of inmates within the penal system is no exception to this arbitrary discretion and specifically the transfer of prisoners from within the general prison population to mental hospitals for the criminally insane have been considered until very recently a purely administrative determination largely devoid of scrutiny. As well as this, the autocratic power of prison administrators in the field of criminal commitment is statutorily authorised in the vast majority of US states. There have been recent advances in the legal rights of the mentally ill however the statutory law of criminal commitment has generally lagged far behind; and criminal commitment procedures in most states remain a matter of administrative discretion or convenience. In Arkansas for example when a prison staff physician ascertains that a prisoner is mentally ill and certifies this finding to the warden of the prison, it becomes the wardens duty to transfer that prisoner to the state hospital until 'reason [is] restored' (Arkansas Statute, 1971).

In common with previous discussion in the Irish context, US literature also discusses whether or not commitment to a mental institution curtails the prisoners' physical liberty because it may extend the length of his incarceration. Look notes that in Baxstrom vs. Herald the Supreme Court held that a transferred prisoner cannot be confined in a mental institution beyond the end of a prison sentence unless he is formally committed under a State Civil

Commitment Statute, or similarly protected procedures. Despite this judgement, the prisoner may still lose the opportunity through the parole and good time systems employed by state prisons in the US. In some states, Look notes parole is statutorily unavailable to prisoners who have been committed, for instance in New Jersey. Even when parole is not statutorily precluded parole boards are extremely reluctant to grant parole to committed prisoners and the practical result is the same as if there was a statutory preclusion. In Arizona for example the transferred prisoner loses certain good time benefits. The lost opportunity for parole may of itself constitute a sufficient deprivation of liberty to implicate findings of due process and the question of human rights arises. The Supreme Court has held that an individual must be afforded due process prior to the revocation of parole or probation. More specifically other courts have held that the denial of parole is a sufficient deprivation of liberty to warrant observance of due process in parole determinations. Look notes that since committed prisoners lose the opportunity for early release through parole criminal commitment should be considered so grievous a loss as to warrant implication of the due process clause.

Civil commitment of a prisoner who is already confined in a mental institution is little more than a rubber-stamp proceeding despite the application of many rigorous procedural safeguards. The civil commitment determination, whether made by a jury or judge hinges almost always exclusively on the expert psychiatric testimony. The psychiatrist's determination is likely to be a foregone conclusion based on his opinion that a currently committed prisoner must be mentally ill. Therefore the administrative decision of prison staff initially to commit a prisoner to a mental institution which was originally meant to last only as long as the sentence, may lead to a much longer period of confinement than the sentence, and in many instances the prisoner remains committed for the rest of his life.

In Schuster vs Herald it states:

'there is repetitive evidence that once a patient has remained in a large mental hospital for two years or more he is quite unlikely to leave except by death'.

This is a topic which has aroused much debate in the United States, as in the UK and Ireland. Bean 2008 notes that mental health legislation uses detention to solve what is essentially a socio-legal-medical problem. It provides detention through an alternative legal system than prison with minimal restrictions or formal procedural rules, and without the usual sets of rights granted to offenders within criminal justice. It solves many of the problems of dealing with mentally disordered offenders using professional medical personal

Involuntary commitment derives ultimately from moral and social considerations not medical ones. A patient may be detained in order to receive treatment, but the detention itself is the vehicle by which treatment is provided. Moreover, considerations that determine commitment, danger to self or others, are also moral and social, and what constitutes an acceptable or unacceptable risk is morally and socially driven. Risks are not the same today as they were yesterday and risks will be different tomorrow. Changing the social situation and what is acceptable behaviour changes the nature of risk in this context.

3.7 Developments in New Zealand – non-completion of treatment

Non-completion of medical treatment is a common occurrence in prisons; such non-completion compromises service cost efficiency; and impacts adversely on both staff and service users' morale; it also may limit the effectiveness of therapy. McMurran and Ward, Queensland researchers, (2010) have stated that attention has to be paid to enhancing an offender's readiness for treatment and developing and maintaining their engagement. They state that research and practice in offender treatment readiness and engagement need to be driven in four major ways. Firstly, the construction of models of engagement that is theoretically based and empirically evidenced that can underpin assessments and treatments. Secondly, there needs to be the development of psychometrically robust assessment of treatment readiness and motivational engagement that can be used to select offenders for treatment or measure change over time. Thirdly, the design, implementation and evaluation of pre-treatment preparation procedures need to be undertaken that can promote treatment engagement and completion. Finally, they advocate the development of strategies that address barriers to engagement as an integral part of treatment.

The authors of this New Zealand study note that non-completion of treatment is also a common occurrence in non-prison populations as well as prison populations and it is undoubtedly a problem both for service users themselves and service providers. An analysis of psychotherapy dropout showed a mean non-completion rate of 47% indicating that a number of participants are not sufficiently engaged in the process of behaviour change (Wierzbicki and Pekarik 1993). Hansen et al (2002) systematically reviewed randomised controlled trials that reported treatment outcomes in terms of the percentage of clients who showed clinically significant improvement. They found that 13 sessions were associated with clinically significant improvement in 58-67% of clients' treatment which is broadly consistent with studies of psychotherapy outcome in other jurisdictions. Therefore in order to substantially benefit from therapy it appears necessary to achieve a certain number of sessions attended. However a finding of the Hansen et al study is that a third of psychotherapy clients only receive one session and the median number of sessions attended is just three.

McMurran and Thedosi (2007) note in their review of offender treatment that re-offending was higher for those who did not complete treatment than for those who were not offered treatment even though the two groups were likely to be of similar risk for re-offending. Early termination of therapy is associated with reduced likelihood of the client attaining clinically significant improvement. Also, with offenders, treatment non-completion might lead to worse outcomes in terms of increased risks to the community and less individual benefits than if treatment had not been undertaken in the first place.

With this in mind the question of how to increase engagement in treatment and reduce rates of treatment non-completion must be asked. Motivation can be a factor as McMurran and Ward (2010) note. They note there is the issue of whether to view an individual's motivation for treatment as a selection criterion, that is, to treat only those individuals who are sufficiently motivated to enter into a treatment programme; or alternatively, to attempt to instil a desire for treatment in otherwise unmotivated individuals. Another option is to have complete disregard for offender's motivation for treatment which may equate to coercion into treatment, and coercion does not lead to the best treatment outcomes. Encouraging offenders to engage in treatment and developing treatment approaches to better suit offenders needs are better ways of working but even so there will be some offenders who remain unmotivated for treatment. Having said that respecting offenders' right to autonomy and ability to make decisions for themselves is ethically more defensible than insisting they partake in treatment programmes. Taking treatment readiness and motivation seriously makes sense both from pragmatic and ethical perspectives. In the Irish context, it is up to the individual offender entirely whether he will participate in treatment programmes as it is an entirely voluntary facility.

3.8 Concluding Comments

In this chapter outlining research in other jurisdictions I have identified key topics that have come up in some of the main English speaking countries of the world, including the United Kingdom, the United States and New Zealand. Throughout the chapter I have tried to refer to how the international research impacts on the Irish context in terms of Irish law, procedures and practices.

The influence of modern forensic psychology on psychiatry is discussed in research conducted in the United Kingdom. This includes a discussion of the terms "dangerous and severely personality disorderd" (DSPD), psychopathic, and the difference between these terms and the commonly understood mental illnesses that occur in society such as schizophrenia.

A brief overview of prison policy in the UK and USA follows this and research in both countries draws upon the impact of economics on how society thinks about rehabilitation and punitive measures for offenders.

The section on the Victorian era historical context is common to most countries in the western world, as the rise of institutionalisation in mental hospitals for the insane were an attempt to rid society of the mentally ill while keeping them safe; and this was often done in a criminal justice context as those who were mentally unfit were often seen as criminally insane because of socially exclusionary behaviours that brought them to police attention.

Recent developments in mental health law follows this discussion and it is observed by Peay

(2003) that mental health law is now largely applied by non-lawyers. Old-fashioned treatments and their modern counterparts are discussed in relation to degrading treatments such as ECT and the modern revolution of pharmacology which appears to bring a good quality of life to most patients.

A discussion on the role of prison administrators in relation to making very significant decisions to commit offenders to mental hospitals takes place in the United States context, and the very significant impact this will have on whether or not they will be eventually released following civil commitment.

Finally I have drawn on New Zealand research into the effects of non-completion of psychotherapeutic treatment in relation to risks for re-offending, and made reference to the Irish procedural context in relation to this.

The next Chapter will be the outcome of my findings using original research data compiled by interviewing a number of professionals involved in both mental health and criminal justice. This will draw upon observations from Garda members, prison psychologist, consultant psychiatrist, social worker, barrister, Chief Executives of voluntary mental health charity and Mental Health Commission and two carers of a person found not guilty but insane under the Criminal Law Insanity Act 2006.

Chapter Four: Research Findings

4.1 Introduction

This chapter focuses on presenting the findings obtained during the course of the research for this study. This includes semi-structured interviews, seven of which were conducted with professionals involved in mental health or criminal justice, and two carers. In this chapter I will review the research questions highlighted for discussion in Chapter One and refer to the research that I have conducted. The quotes which will be used in this chapter are from my notes which are not verbatim representations of what was said at interview.

4.2 Limitations

The subjects in my study, most of whom have requested not to be named, cannot be considered fully representative of all views which could be held by professionals or organisations who may be involved in the sector. This is because of the personal nature of their experience and the subjectivity of the semi-structured interview structure. It is also because of the short time frame involved in conducting this study which limited the number of professionals I could interview and the limit placed upon the researcher by the total word count of fifteen thousand words for a complete overview of the topic under review. However, I believe that this chapter does deliver a keen insight into very relevant research questions brought up by the topic of this dissertation as outlined in Chapter One.

4.3 Research Question Number One: What are the links between An Garda Siochana and the mental health services?

An Garda Siochana have a role in keeping the public safe, preventing crime and in keeping the peace, therefore they are often asked to intervene when a person is mentally ill and in need of hospitalisation, or when a mentally ill person commits crime as a result of their illness or otherwise.

The Executive Director of Shine – Supporting People Affected by Mental Ill health, a charity funded by the HSE, indicated in relation to this question that in terms of An Garda Siochana, most experience are derived from "on the street activities" and that Gardaí are involved in mental health matters where family members of a person with a mental health problem particularly call Garda when it comes to coping with the illness and committing the person to hospital. He noted that involuntary admissions occurred particularly under the Mental Health 1945 Act where Gardaí escorted people to a hospital for admission, but under the Mental Health Act 2001 there is less Garda involvement. When asked how Gardaí, in his experience, handle mental health matters, he stated that Gardaí by and large handle things fairly well and this is particularly noticeable with older, more experienced Gardaí who have learned on the job how to deal with these incidences. He did point out however, that very little training is given to Gardaí on the issue of mental ill health and this is an area of deficit that needs to be corrected, in his view.

In contrast to this view, the carers interviewed in relation to this study, were parents of a person with schizophrenia who committed a serious crime and was found not guilty by reason of insanity under the 2006 Criminal Law Insanity Act. Their comments on their first experience of Gardaí in relation to the crime and arrest were that "the Gardaí and the police were so nice to us and when we went to see him [their son] the next night, every Garda member could see he was very ill." They said "the care we got from them [the Gardaí] was amazing."

In relation to training for Garda members on mental health matters, the Barr Tribunal investigated the facts and circumstances surrounding the fatal shooting of John Carthy at Abbeylara in 2000. They made a number of recommendations in relation to partnership between An Garda Siochana and the mental health services. They recommended Garda training in mental illness and siege situations, ensuring an adequate number of psychologists are employed by the state to provide the service of expert assistance in siege situations. They recommended the training of these psychologists in negotiation strategies and establishing formal working relationships between An Garda Siochana and state psychologists. In recent times An Garda Siochana has implemented the recommendations in relation to training in mental illness in siege situations: trained on-scene commanders of Superintendent rank and some at Inspector rank are now in every Garda region. All have received training in controlling siege situations as well as training in mental illness. In addition trained Garda hostage negotiators are now available in each Garda region to support the on-scene commander. A number of sieges, for example Gort, have ended peacefully due to the changes made (Quilter, 2009).

A Garda Inspector with an extensive background in inner city community policing who I interviewed in relation to mental health said that "the Mental Health Act 2001 changed everything". In relation to his own training, the Inspector mentioned that he got training in Templemore as part of the original mental health act training which included the Mental

Health Act 2001. He noted that An Garda Siochana work with medical professionals and the medical boards train their people appropriately also. He stated that the "Gardaí and Sergeants who currently work on the beat would have much more training than the older Gardaí…the guards [who deal with mental illnesses now] are very competent and seem to have good insight".

In my own experience of working within An Garda Siochana, I would say that Gardaí are very well trained to deal with every situation they find themselves in, and this includes dealing with mental health issues of members of the public and criminal behaviour. I have found that many Gardaí are less willing to talk about mental health issues than they might be, and this could be addressed through awareness raising activities and facilitated workshops on mental health.

4.4 Research Question Number Two: What are the links between the courts and the Central Mental Hospital?

The Central Mental Hospital is a designated centre under the legislation so that many criminals with mental illnesses are committed there. Most of the patients who stay in the Central Mental Hospital have a criminal background and come in through the court system.

A social worker in the Central Mental Hospital who I interviewed has been working nearly eight years in her role, and she says "it is always evolving and in constant revolution". She notes that there is an evolution rather than a revolution and there are political directive changes: in the last ten years there have been two serious pieces of legislation to impact the sector (Mental Health Act 2001 and Criminal Law Insanity Act 2006) and the Mental Health Inspectorate was also set up. The Irish Advocacy Network came to the Central Mental Hospital in 2005. These are peer support workers who advocate on behalf of the in-patients in the hospital and also encourage them to advocate for themselves. A Carers Group was also established in 2003.

The social worker notes that there are a number of different types of people who come into the hospital as in-patients, many of whom would come in through the courts and legal processes. There are some detained under the Mental Health Act 2001 with no convictions. The local services would have found these people difficult to cope with as they may have serious behavioural, social or psychological problems. They have access to all the tribunals and reviews allowed under the Mental Health Act. There are also people who are remanded in custody who appear too ill to be in prison. They are not convicted yet, but they may be committed to hospital rather than prison. She notes that they divert people back to local services who have committed petty crime from Cloverhill. There are also people with sentences who become ill in prison; they would be serving reasonably long or life sentences. They come to the Central Mental Hospital for a period of time for treatment before going back to prison. A couple of people serving life sentences, she notes, may spent the entirety of their sentence in the Central Mental Hospital because they are too ill to go back to prison. There are also a group who were found not guilty by reason of insanity under the Criminal Law Insanity Act 2006. The Central Mental Hospital is the only designated centre where this group of patients can be accommodated under the terms of the 2006 Act.

The group found not guilty but insane, the social worker says, are different from other in-patients. They would be from a range of backgrounds, some from professional backgrounds. She indicated that there is not a class system as such but the not guilty by reason of insanity cohort would be white collar rather than blue collar. It demonstrates that mental illness crosses the spectrum of backgrounds. The social worker indicates that persons found not guilty by reason of insanity "…are in a strange place. There is a sense of loss for the person killed and also fractured relationships [with family]". She indicates that it is a very complex thing to help people work things through and it requires a multi-disciplinary team to help these people work through their problems and achieve any level of recovery. She notes that there are five pillars of care within the Central Mental Hospital: physical health; mental health wellness; drug and alcohol issues; harmful behaviours and also psychiatric issues. Everyone has a care plan which focuses on all five pillars. There is a key worker for each person within the multi-disciplinary team.

The carers who I spoke to who indicated that their son came into the Central Mental Hospital through the courts said that he was one of the first offenders to be found not guilty by reason of insanity under the 2006 Act. They said "this was new to the judge and the DPP barrister walked the judge through it….he has a review board meeting every six months and degrees of leave are approved by the justice department. The DPP barrister really led the defence to a conclusion." One thing they indicated that they are particularly concerned about is that the Criminal Law Insanity Act 2006 does not provide for conditional release. Nobody in the Central Mental Hospital under the terms of this Act has been released for this reason. The carers group of which they are members has been lobbying for amendments to the Act which are currently going through the Dáil. They note that there is no care in the community as such, as envisaged under A Vision for Change, for example, so they anticipate there will be a delay clearing the backlog of persons found not guilty by reason of insanity who may be recommended for release into the community if conditions are applied.

A barrister I spoke to indicated that the stakes are very high for criminal offenders using insanity as a defence, and for this reason the numbers of defendants claiming insanity are very small. A person who committed an act while insane, may convince a judge that he has regained sanity and be released from court a free man, although found not guilty but insane at the time of the act. The barrister knew of two cases where this had happened. On the other hand there could be a commitment to the Central Mental Hospital for an indeterminate length with no probability of release, if the person was found still to be insane by the court.

The barrister also mentioned a stigma about mental illness which exists in Irish society and in communities where offenders would live which would lead a criminal offender to prefer a prison sentence than commitment in a hospital. He noted that criminals liked the certainty of a prison sentence with credit for good time behaviour and disliked the uncertainty of open-ended commitment to a hospital and the administration of medical treatment which goes along with that. He mentioned that it would be quite common for a jury not to hear about a mental illness but for a judge to hear it as a mitigating factor when deciding on sentence in an attempt to shorten the sentence length.

I also met with a consultant psychiatrist who works in the Central Mental Hospital as part of the Prison In-reach and Court Liaison Service. He indicates that there are ten times as many prisoners with major mental illnesses in prisons than there are individuals with major mental illnesses in the community. He notes that people with mental illnesses are more likely to be arrested than a person without a mental illness for the same crime, shoplifting for example. They are more likely to get caught. The offenders may be confused, bewildered or paranoid for example and they are not as likely to respond appropriately to Gardaí. He notes that it is difficult for Gardaí to decide if someone is mentally ill or intoxicated.

4.5   Research Question Three: The criminalisation of persons with mental illnesses

An Garda Siochana do not have much discretion in relation to arrest when a crime is committed even if the perpetrator appears to be mentally ill, therefore there is a tendency for mentally ill persons who commit minor offences to be criminalised.

The consultant psychiatrist I spoke to indicated that prisoners with major mental illnesses do not get bail. They may be homeless, have no money and have lost contact with family members. Therefore they are put in prison or the mental hospital. He notes that there has been in general a move towards community care in the last thirty or forty years in western countries. The same thing happens in other western countries, he notes: hospitals are closed down, but there is less community based care available; there are constant budget cuts and there is no accommodation provided for mentally ill persons. He notes that for a person with a mental illness, the service is delivered by catchment areas, but for a person who becomes homeless this becomes more difficult as they move out of catchment areas where they had been living. "You need to be living in an area for some three months before you can access the service, and it is very difficult to hold down a job and accommodation [while mentally ill]" he says.

Most of the people I interviewed did indicate that in their view in a lot of cases people with mental illnesses did end up in prison, criminalised. One individual noted that there is an essential difference between commitment and incarceration for mentally ill offenders and persons who have no criminal background. He notes that there is essentially a difference of crime, being found guilty, and that you can be mentally ill and have a criminal conviction, sentenced to serve time under punishment. There are people who end up in prison who have committed a crime while mentally ill and he would argue that they should not be there.

In mental health services people are committed under the Mental Health Act 2001 because they are a danger to themselves or others. There are clearly defined procedures in place for commitment. Also there is a comprehensive system regarding detention beyond 21 days in terms of Mental Health Tribunals.

The barrister I interviewed indicated that yes, people with mental illnesses do end up in prison. He said that mental illnesses are not necessarily detected and that people suspected of a crime should have a psychiatric evaluation. He says "the law might be there but it is not applied as skilfully as it might be". He said that not enough attention is paid to people's mental health when they are being charged with a criminal offence and there can be hardened criminals committing crimes. He indicated that ego can also play a role in the courtroom. He gave an example where two women gave evidence against a man who had attacked and raped them and they made terrible witnesses. However he acted up in court and the jury was discharged by the judge. When the retrial happened the women gave flawless evidence and the criminal got a life sentence. The barrister indicated that mental health "does not serve criminal law very well....it is there as an instrument but it is not there for direction."

In my experience people who are able to access a high level of support services such as social housing, social benefits, medical care and employment or training support in community based centres are much less likely to ever come to the attention of the Gardai in a criminal matter. People such as these may have experience of being committed to hospital with the help of An Garda Siochana, but more likely they will not have committed crime. The problem for society is that there is not enough support services for people with mental illnesses and therefore they do end up committing low level crimes and becoming criminalised.

4.6 Research Question Number Four: What is the difference for society between retribution for a crime and rehabilitation? Does it make a difference in practice?

Criminal sanctions such as prison within a society are used for punishment and to a certain extent as society's retribution for a crime committed. The question of whether a criminal can be rehabilitated while in prison; or a criminal with a mental illness can achieve recovery while committed to a hospital are complex and varied.

I spoke to the Chief Executive of the Mental Health Commission, Mr. Hugh Kane.
Hugh Kane indicated to me at interview that the regulations about prison are very clear. "The mental health service has less of an emphasis on in-patient care and if you are treated at home in the community there would be less problems." He points out that "the fact is, they [the state] can lock you up, keep you there, and medicate you against your will if you are not well". He does note that "there are lots of other options besides prisons; there is restorative justice, community support and community services. For certain groups of people the bar is very low for prison and for other groups the bar is very high. People can be rehabilitated. If you look at proportions of lower socio-economic backgrounds in prison, travellers for instance get put in prison for stealing clothes. They are seen by the courts to be very mobile and are not given bail for that reason." In relation to serious crime, he points out that there are some people who are "just bad and the deprivation of liberty is the punishment…there should be some engagement with the person to allow them reflect on that." In relation to prison itself, he says that "to a lot of us, who have never experienced prison, slopping out, for instance, it's a fair penalty…it's quite a punishment."

Mr. Kane goes on to say that if you have a mental illness, recovery and rehabilitation may apply, usually for a low level crime. The low level nature of most crimes committed by mentally ill persons is backed up by the Garda Inspector I spoke to and also Director of Shine. I would say that there appears to be a public perception that persons with major mental illnesses, for example schizophrenia, are violent to a greater extent than persons without a mental illness but the facts do not back up this perception, and for example says that "the numbers of persons with mental illnesses who commit crime are smaller than you might think".

There is a question to be asked about criminals with mental illnesses: is it mental illness that causes criminality or does criminal behaviour cause mental illness. Drug addiction and alcohol abuse is a vicious cycle which is a contributory cause to emotional disturbance among people in prisons who often end up in hospital. Hugh Kane points out that we need to deal with people with mental health problems, "they should not be locked up without recovery…Some people do need to be locked up to keep [society] safe, but there are still people who recover…the stigma of mental illness frightens people off."

The prison psychologist in Mountjoy who I spoke to said in relation to rehabilitation and retribution that "society needs to feel it is punishing people…as psychologists, we feel that punishment should decrease the behaviour…in fact, imprisonment makes you more likely to re-offend….it is a governor's role to manage offenders in prison, not to make them fit for release." She indicates that there is a clash of cultures "for the offender, prison is like a rite of passage not a punishment".

In answer to the question do prisoners ultimately have the final say on whether they will accept efforts to rehabilitate, she said that as prison staff they have to engage or the prisoners will re-offend, and in terms of difficulties there are large numbers of people with personality disorders in prison and they are particularly difficult to engage with.

In my own view, low level criminals learn more about criminal behaviour in prison and they increase their criminal contacts in prison, therefore they will be more likely to re-offend upon release. Whether people who commit crimes while mentally ill do actually end up in prison is a question which I put to my interview subjects and the people I interviewed all indicated that yes, they do. There is certainly recovery that is possible for most people within a mental health setting for people who commit crime with mental illnesses, the question for society is does it want retribution for the crime or rehabilitation for the individual.

4.7 Research Question Number Five: Discussion of competency to stand trial for mentally ill offenders; what is the role of medication in restoring competency?

There are occasions when a very serious crime is committed by a person suffering an acute episode of mental illness, where he may act out on delusions or voices in his head and commit murder, for example. The question of competency to stand trial arises in such instances.

The consultant psychiatrist in the Central Mental Hospital, who I spoke to, said in relation to competency to stand trial, "on any given day, it wouldn't really matter if a person was fit to be tried, the best steps [to restore competency] are appropriate care and treatment. The case must be appropriate." He added that "beds in Dundrum should not be blocked with minor issues". I would infer from this that as an acute in-patient facility for seriously ill persons, competency to stand trial in the Central Mental Hospital is therefore a matter of the greatest severity and the nature of the crimes would indicate this also.

In relation to fitness to be tried, a report is prepared for the court voluntarily or on request from the consultant psychiatrist with a detailed psychiatric history. This diagnoses fitness to be tried and it should include a workable plan whether he is put in custody or granted bail. There are sometimes non-custodial disposals, such as offering an offender a bed in a hospital with bail conditions about medication, substance abuse and agreement to be transported by Gardaí. He points out that the prison in-reach service does not want to be diverting people out of prisons who pose a significant risk.

The prison in reach and court diversion service deal with many stakeholders to get a better picture and help the Gardaí and the court make the most informed decisions. He points out that the relationship with Gardaí is excellent and that the judges welcome diversion as well. The prison in-reach service won a Healthcare Award in 2009. The service has been well received and it was established under the early implementation of a recommendation of the mental health policy document A Vision for Change, published in 2006.

In relation to the potential gaps in the system for treating mentally ill offenders, the psychiatrist I spoke with points out that the diversion system is there for the great majority of prisoners and the gaps "might be limited resources for homeless people…they are massively under-resourced and the shelter homes for the homeless have huge needs… the access to psychiatric beds when you're homeless can be more difficult than when you're not homeless." He added that the homeless can be most severely in need but they don't have the access when they are not in the catchment area. "More beds in Dundrum could be provided and there is a need for more local secure units – St. Brendan's on the north side of Dublin have a small number." He pointed out that there is a shortage of locked wards in Ireland, referring to the fact that in the 1960s there were 30,000 beds for psychiatric patients, usually with fewer problems than today. Now there are less than 3000 beds for psychiatric patients and the services have not been provided in the community and there is downward pressure on mental health budgets.

In relation to medication's role in restoring competency to stand trial I would say that in my experience most people with mental illnesses who commit serious crime may have been non-compliant with medication at the time of committing the act, and that most people can be restored to competency if they are treated in hospital following the episode. Thereafter they can receive an appropriate sentence. Sometimes a serious crime can be committed by someone with no history of mental illness but a judge can determine that they were mentally ill at the time and commit them to serve out a sentence in the Central Mental Hospital on advice from a psychiatrist.

4.8   Research Question Number Six: What about Government Policy on Mental Health, "A Vision for Change", four years after publication, in the midst of a very severe recession?

One of the main tenets of A Vision for Change was the relocation of the Central Mental Hospital in Dundrum to a new site. The proposed site which the government have been considering for a long time was on the site of the proposed super-prison to be built at Thornton Hall. The carers I spoke with in the course of this study, said that their group, the Carers Group of the Central Mental Hospital had lobbied the government for a long time, not to put the Central Mental Hospital onto the site of a prison. That was one of their major issues with A Vision for Change, the location of the hospital. In spite of this, the carers indicated to me that there has been a huge improvement in recent times in the Central Mental Hospital since A Vision for Change had been conceptualised. They say that Harry Kennedy, Clinical Director of the Central Mental Hospital is a driving force behind the change.

In the Central Mental Hospital there is a patient forum which meets every two weeks, they campaign in their own right. They are coordinated by the Irish Advocacy Network, who has two representatives in the hospital. They encourage the patients to advocate on their own behalf.

The consultant psychiatrist I spoke with indicated that the court diversion process and prison in-reach service with which he is involved came about as a result of the first phase of implementation of A Vision for Change. He points out that the closure of beds in hospitals can be a good thing, but only if there is enough investment in community resources and accommodation for persons with mental illnesses. Unfortunately, he says the money which may have been available when A Vision for Change was being conceptualised, has disappeared and what is left is not being put into community resources. In relation to housing, supported housing policy gives priority to single mothers, and single men with mental illnesses or brain injury are not given priority. He points out that housing, health and justice have three different budgets within the Irish government context and that there is no coherent strategy to deliver a joined-up solution to improving the lives of people affected by mental ill health. "You could get a better life for people if there was a coherent strategy," he says.

A Vision for Change is a very good there is very slow implementation because of resources to date.

The barrister I spoke to said that with twenty-first century thinking "there should be in every province a facility devoid of institutional manifestations where people with mental illnesses can be assessed in a gentle constructive way…sending the vast majority of people to prisons is crazy…psychiatry or psychology can play a much bigger part".

I would suggest that resourcing care in the community and providing social accommodation for mentally ill persons must happen in tandem with closing down unfit for purpose mental hospitals as envisaged in A Vision for Change. However to date this has not happened. People have been transferred from old hospitals to psychiatric wings of general hospitals rather than be accommodated and supported in communities and this is not in the spirit or letter of the policy document that was published in 2006, but of course public finances are of primary concern.

4.9   Concluding Comments

During the course of this study, carrying out the interviews with the professionals and carers I gained a deep insight into topics that generally would not come up in the literature. Interviewees, because they were not being taped, and because I had agreed not to disclose their names in many cases, were very open with me and expressed their views freely.   In general there is a stigma around mental illness in Irish as in other societies, and this too was evident in the interviews that I undertook. People are more reluctant to talk about mental illness than perhaps other types of disability, or indeed many of the other of the nine protected grounds under equality legislation.   The interviews, semi-structured as they were, are by design very subjective in nature.

I agree with the barrister who indicated that criminals are reluctant to have evidence of mental illness put before the jury because they are afraid of being stigmatised and subjected to unwanted medical treatment in hospital. However I am quite sure, as he indicated, that psychiatric evidence is heard in private by the judge to determine sentence. In most of these cases after conviction, the criminal is put into prison even though he has a documented mental illness, which seems to verify one of my research questions 'do people with mental illnesses end up in prison?'

The carers and mental health Chief Executives who I interviewed were convinced that placing the new Central Mental Hospital on the site of the new prison at Thornton Hall would be a mistake. Their thinking was that in the public's view it would portray people with mental illnesses in the same way as criminals. However the prison psychologist who I spoke to did not appear to have a problem with this, as she indicated both prisoners and the mentally ill are equally stigmatised by society anyway. I would not be of this view, and I think that the way people with mental illnesses are portrayed in society and in the media is very important.

I think that more resources should be put into looking after the mental health needs of the homeless, having spoken to the consultant psychiatrist at the Central Mental Hospital who revealed that by virtue of homelessness many people can be excluded from accessing services. Often it is left to charities and religious orders to provide hot meals during the day for homeless people and their resources available to see to medical attention would be very limited. There are some services such as Usher's Island which have psychiatric nurses and a social worker onsite, but I believe due to resource cuts they are no longer in a position to provide hot meals.

In the concluding chapter I will review the study and draw conclusions where appropriate and look into areas for further study which may be related to the topic linking mental health to criminal justice. I hope that my research will prove to be a valuable resource for anyone with an interest in mental health and criminality and professionals who may be involved in either field.

Chapter Five: Summary, Conclusions and Recommendations

5.1 Summary

In this study I have summarised the main most common types of mental illnesses that occur in society and the main two pieces of legislation that have been introduced in the last ten years that impact upon people with mental illnesses: The Mental Health Act 2001 and the Criminal Law (Insanity) Act 2006. I noted in particular the significant stigma attached to mental illness that exists in Irish society and particularly within the family of a person with mental illness which is compounded when involuntary admissions to a hospital happen under the 2001 Act, particularly when there is Garda involvement.

I outlined how homelessness impacts on mental illness and that more homeless people have mental illnesses than the general population. Homelessness and crime are also inextricably linked as numerous studies have suggested that being homeless increases significantly the chances of individuals entering the criminal justice system, and often not being released on bail. I outlined how case management is a process whereby An Garda Siochana manages the criminal behaviour of juveniles, some of whom may have aged out having turned eighteen years old and may be at risk of homelessness or mental ill health due to a difficult background.

I outlined how diversion takes place between the prison system and mental health services and how this helps persons with mental illnesses from staying in the prison system, at least for a time. I spoke about the pharmaceutical revolution which has impacted the treatment of persons with mental illnesses over the last number of decades, whereby psychoactive drugs are prescribed to restore competency. Most mental health service users have the experience of being medicated for their problems and many have great success in leading normal lives as a result of this intervention.

I noted how women make up 5% of the prison population worldwide and how this is also true in the Irish context. Most of the research that has been carried out has focussed on male prisoners and as a result the impact of prison on women has not been studied particularly extensively in the literature. A consistent picture of poverty, marginalisation, and deprivation constitutes the basis of the female custodial population in prisons. There is a pattern of abuse, drug addiction, poverty and unemployment together with psychological disturbances in women prisoners.

A Vision for Change is the pre-recession Government policy on mental health published in 2006 when it appeared that the resources could be made available over the ten year timeframe of the document to actually implement this far reaching policy in Ireland. As a result of inspections old hospitals and unsuitable wards in hospitals are being closed to new patients and are being closed down. However, unlike the vision for the future in the policy document, the people who have been institutionalised by their mental illness have not been accommodated in supported housing in the community, they have rather been moved to different wings of general hospitals and remain institutionalised.

As I mentioned, homelessness is a big issue for the mentally ill, and often people stay in hospitals because they have nowhere else to go. Getting the resources and services available in the community can be a hard battle to fight, particularly when you are unwell.

In Chapter Three I commented on UK research which indicated that dangerous and severely personality disordered (DSPD) persons populate prisons and it is a much argued debate as to whether or not they can benefit from a stay in a psychiatric hospital. I noted the significant differences between major mental illnesses and the DSPD label for offenders who essentially use different services within the prison system.

I noted that in North America and much of Europe modern prison policies have been characterised by swings from rehabilitative to punitive measures and back again. Public attitudes to crime and justice may reflect socio-economic dynamics of a given culture, and consequently attempts to assess attitudes may not always yield consistently accurate measures of public beliefs.

I mentioned that the modern mental health system has its roots in the Victorian world view because they were urged to help the "mad" and "eccentric" in society. In relation to mental health law, I noted that mental health was now largely applied by non-lawyers and that medical professionals are given the primary responsibility and the powers to decide who should and who should not be admitted to hospital and the treatment to be provided.

I noted that some commentators argue that the conditions for civil commitment have never provided adequate justification for commitment, for as Thomas Szasz observes "mental illness is a myth and hospitalisation is a modern form of state controlled warfare". I would not agree with this commentator as I believe mental illness is very real and limited and legally robust justifications must and do exist for civil commitment under the relevant legislation.

I noted that in US research prison administrators have historically exercised what many legal scholars call autocratic discretion in relation to determining whether or not a prisoner should be committed to a psychiatric institution during their sentence or recommending that they stay in such an institution beyond the period of when their sentence would end if it is medically considered that the person is unfit for release in society.

I noted the New Zealand study which indicated that non-completion of medical treatment is common occurrence in prisons, and it limits the effectiveness of therapy, usually leading to reoffending.

In Chapter Four I introduced the research of the semi-structured interviews that I undertook during the investigation of this study and I examined and discussed the research questions that I set for myself in Chapter One.

The next section of this Chapter will set out the conclusions and recommendations that I have reached, and suggest ways that a future researcher might continue to investigate the important topics that I have raised in this study.

5.2   Conclusions and Recommendations

In the Report of the Joint Working Group on Mental Health Services and the Police published in 2009 and referred to in Chapter One of this study, the importance of training is stressed by the stakeholders who are involved in consulting in this report.

"All the participant groups stressed the need for all Gardaí to get training in aspects of mental health and mental illness, to equip them to deal with crisis situations. The participants described the need for particular skills and knowledge; service users and family were particularly clear that Gardaí should meet and learn directly from people who have experienced mental health problems and from their families".

Gardaí have a duty to protect the citizens of the state and uphold and enforce law and order. They are the only agency who is immediately available day or night to respond to crises in the community, including those involving psychiatric patients. All of the professionals I spoke to indicate that the Gardaí are very professional in how they carry out their work on behalf of those members of society with mental illnesses, however the view was expressed that perhaps they are not trained adequately to deal with mental illness in members of the public.

My own view, having worked with An Garda Siochana for three years in my current role as Higher Executive Officer in the Dublin Metropolitan Region is that An Garda Siochana are a very professional police force who are very well trained to deal with people and any crisis they face in the community or elsewhere. There have been mistakes made in the past such as Abbeylara in 2000 but the recommendations that came out of that inquiry have been implemented to a very great extent and An Garda Siochana have learned from that experience.

A Memorandum of Understanding between An Garda Siochana and the Health Service Executive was developed and signed by Garda Commissioner Fachtna Murphy and Chief Executive Officer of the HSE Mr. Cathal McGee on 15th September 2010. One of the aims is to include the development of the formal liaison systems between the mental health services and An Garda Siochana as recommended in the Joint Working Group report. Another key goal was to establish a good working relationship between the mental health service and An Garda Siochana in respect of collaboration in addressing the needs of persons with mental ill health.

One of the other recommendations on the Joint Working Group report is the development of a training programme which facilitates members of An Garda Siochana in recognising and responding appropriately to people with mental illness in crisis and providing information on community and social services. Such a programme should include involvement of service users, families and representatives from the mental health and social services and the training should be included in the overall training for new Garda recruits, and also included in ongoing professional programmes for members of An Garda Siochana.

Training on mental health has been provided to Garda recruits in Templemore by the national organisation SHINE – Supporting People Affected by Mental ill Health in recent years. This training has involved both service users and professionals involved in coordinating the needs of mental health service users and their families. There is also specific module on mental health contained in probationer Gardaí training, but I was unable to examine this for the purpose of this study.

One of the conclusions that must inevitably be drawn as a result of this study is that people with mental illnesses who have committed crime do end up in prison. A greater proportion of prisoners have mental illnesses than those in the general population and there are only 82 in patient beds in the Central Mental Hospital, placed against a backdrop of several thousand prison spaces throughout the country, so at any given time there must inevitably be people with mental illnesses, or acute psychotic or depressive symptoms, in the prison population.

This study explores the links between mental health and the criminal justice system. There are very few studies of this type but exploring further the issues of social exclusion and poverty and its impact on criminality would be an interesting topic to explore for another researcher. The intergenerational nature of many families who are beneficiaries of welfare whose family members end up involved in crime would be an interesting topic to explore.

The twin topics of mental disorder and substance abuse have not been explored in detail in this study, but there is a definite link. In exploring the research literature on mental illness and crime one would think that researchers are primarily interested in the links to violent crime and particularly in the links with schizophrenia of which there are countless studies. There is nothing substantial in the research literature for instance on mental illness and burglary, shoplifting, fraud, criminal damage and dishonestly handling stolen property (Bean, 2009). However, typically these are the types of crimes together with public order offences which the professionals I interviewed indicated that people with mental illnesses commit, who come before the law courts.

There is a reluctance to treat patients with substance abuse problems and mental illnesses as they have a detrimental effect on hospitals. The consultant psychiatrist I spoke with indicated that the diversion programme he is involved in would not be an option for such an offender. Studies on substance abuse and mental illness, where they exist, concentrate more on the substance abuse than the mental illness.

To produce a more balanced literature on mental health and criminal justice we need a greater level of interest from criminologists, especially sociologists able to promote studies dealing with the mentally ill within the community, including the impact of criminal justice programmes on mental disorder. There is also a dearth of literature on the experience of the mentally ill offender in the police station or in inner cities where criminality is rife. The emphasis in linking mental illness and crime should be on the criminal behaviour or on offenders who are mentally ill, rather than the term which is often used 'mentally ill offenders'. The emphasis should be on the criminality not on the mental illness. If we focus on this emphasis we will know more about the links between mental illness and crime and perhaps a more rational set of policy objectives may be developed.

References

Adler, Joanna ed. (2004) <u>Forensic Psychology, Concepts, Debates and Practice</u>, Willan Publishing

Arkansas Statute (1971) 59-415, in Joseph Look, 'Transfer of Prisoners to Mental Institutions' in <u>The Journal of Criminal Law and Criminology</u>, Vol 69 No. 3 (Autumn 1978) pp331-352 Northwestern University

Baxtrom v Herold (1966), 383 US 107 (1966) pp 26-28

Bean, P. (2008), <u>Madness and Crime</u>, Willan Publishing

Bell J., Campbell S., Erikson M. Hogue T, McLean Z., Rust S., and Taylor R (2003) 'An overview: DSPD programme concepts and progress' in A. Lord and L. Rayment (eds) <u>Dangerous and Severe personality Disorder (Issues in Forensic Psychology</u> 4). Leicester: British Psychological Society, Division of Forensic Psychology

Byrne MK, and Howells, K (2002) 'Womens perception of the prison environment: When prison is "the safest place I've ever been"', <u>Psychology of Women Quarterly</u>, 26 (4):351-59

Chiricos, TG. And DeLone MA (1992) 'Labour Surplus and Punishment: A review and assessment of theory and evidence', <u>Social Problems</u>, 39: pp421-46

Connolly, N (2005), 'Ireland to copy Britian's Controversial ASBOs', <u>Sunday Business Post</u> May 08, 2005

Cotton, J (2003), <u>Police Complaints and Discipline: England and Wales, 12 Months to March 2003</u>, Home Office, United Kingdom

Department of Health and Children (2006), <u>A Vision for Change, Report of the Expert Group on Mental Health Policy</u>

Duffy D, Linehan S, Kennedy HG, (2006) 'Psychiatric morbidity in the male sentenced Irish prisons population', <u>Irish Journal of Psychological Medicine</u> 2006; Vol 23 No 2: 54-62.

Dushkind, D.S. (1984), 'Forensic Psychology - a proposed definition' <u>American Journal of Forensic Psychology</u>, 2(4):171-72

Expert Committee (1999), <u>Report of the Expert Committee: Review of the Mental Health Act 1983</u> (Richardson Committeee) London: Department of Health

Feehan, M. and Brown, A (2009), An Garda Siochana, <u>Review and Development of a Garda Case Management Pilot Project</u>, An Garda Siochana in association with Children Acts Advisory Board

Focus Ireland (2007) <u>The Impact of Homelessness</u>, Information Sheet

Freeman, Karen (1998), '<u>Mental Health and the Criminal Justice System</u>', Crime and Justice

Bulletin, Number 38, NSW Bureau of Crime Statistics and Research

Government of Ireland (2001), <u>Mental Health Act 2001</u>, Dublin Stationery Office

Government of Ireland (2006) <u>Criminal Law (Insanity) Act 2006</u>, Dublin Stationery Office

Greenland, C. (1970) <u>Mental Illness and Civil Liberty</u>, Occasional Papers on Social Administration No. 38, Bell

Hansen NB, Lambert MJ and Forman EM (2002) 'The psychotherapy dose-response effect and its implications for treatment delivery services' in <u>Clinical Psychology: Science and Practice</u> 9: 329-343

Hickey, Claire (2002) <u>Crime and Homelessness</u>, Focus Ireland and PACE

Karem (2005) 'Commentary: A Multi-disciplinary Approach to Developing Mental Health Training for Law Enforcement', <u>Journal of the American Academy of Psychiatry and the Law,</u> 33, pp47-49

Kennedy, Harry (2007), <u>The Annotated Mental Health Acts</u>, Blackhall Publishing

Kury, H., and Ferdinand T. (1999) 'Public opinion and punitivity', <u>International Journal of Law and Psychiatry</u>, 22: 373-92

Look, J (1978) 'Transfer of Prisoners to Mental Institutions' in <u>The Journal of Criminal Law</u>

and Criminology, Vol 69 No. 3 (Autumn 1978) pp331-352 Northwestern University

Loucks, Nancy (2004) 'Women in Prison', in Forensic Psychology, Concepts Debates and Practice, by Joanna Adler (ed), Willan Publishing

Maguire M., Morgan R., and Reiner R. (eds) (2002) The Oxford Handbook of Criminology, 3rd Edition. Oxford: Oxford University Press

McGarry, L (1997), 'The Nature of Competency to Stand Trial,' in Ethics of Psychiatry, edited by Rem B Edwards, Prometheus Books, New York

McMurran M, Thedosi E (2007) ' Is treatment non-completion associated with increase reconviction over no treatment? Psychology, Crime and Law 13: 333-343

McMurran M. and Ward, T (2010), 'Treatment Readiness, treatment engagement and behaviour change', in Criminal Behaviour and Mental Health, 20:75-85

Melossi, D. (2000) 'Changing Representations of the Criminal', British Journal of Criminology 40: 296-320

Mental Health Commission / An Garda Siochana (2009), Report of Joint Working Group on Mental Health Services and the Police 2009

Peay, J (2003) Decisions and Dilemmas, Oxford: Hart

Perkins, D and Bishopp D. (2003), 'Dangerous and Severe Personality Disorder and its relationship to sexual offending,' in A. Lord and L. Rayment (eds) <u>Dangerous and Severe presonality Disorder (Issues in Forensic Psychology</u> 4). Leicester: British Psychological Society, Division of Forensic Psychology

Porter, R. (1991) <u>The Faber Book of Madness</u>, London: Faber and Faber.

Quilter, John (2009) An Garda Siochana, Unpublished Dissertation on <u>Joint Garda Mental Health Teams</u>, Institute of Public Administration

Schull, A. (1985) 'A Victorian Alienist: John Connoly FRCP, DCC (1794-1866)' in W.F.Bynum, R. Porter and M. Shepherd (eds) (1985) <u>The Anatomy of Madness, Volume 1:</u> London Tavistock 103-50.

Schuster v Herold (1969) 410 F 2nd 1071 (2nd) 396 US 847

Seymour M and Costello L (2005), <u>'A Study of the Number, Profile and Progression Routes of Homeless Persons before the Court and in Custody'</u>, Centre for Social and Educational Research, DIT Dublin.

Shine (2009) Unpublished <u>Submission to Mental Health Commission on Joint Working Group on Police and Mental Health</u>

Singleton N., Meltzer H. And Gatward R with J. Coid and D. Deasy (1998), <u>Psychiatric morbidity among prisoners</u>: A survey carried out in 1997 by the Social Survey Division of DNS on behalf of the Department of Health, London Office for National Statistics

Sparks R (2000) 'Penal "austerity": the doctrine of less eligibiliity reborn?' in R. Matthews and P. Francis, <u>Prison 2000: An International Perspective on the Current State and Future of Imprisonment</u> London: McMillan

Szasz, T (1960). 'The Myth of Mental Illness', in <u>the American Psychologist</u> 15: 113-18

Wierzbicki M. and Pekarik G (1993), 'A meta-analysis of psychotherapy dropout', in Professional Psychology Research and Practice 24: 190-195